The Ult____

Plant Based Diet Cookbook

More Than 50 Delectable Recipes to Shed Weight, Heal Your Body, and Regain Confidence

Pearl Jones

TABLE OF CONTENTS

INTRODUCTION

A plant-based diet is a diet that includes mainly plants and excludes meat and other animal products. The term "plant-based" does not mean vegetarian or vegan. Plants provide the fuel for any human, regardless of their dietary preferences. This is because humans are omnivores, capable of digesting both plant and animal foodstuffs. Many traditional diets have been plant-based; they include fruits, vegetables, grains, nuts and beans as staple foods without including meat or other animal products at all.

When people look at the list of foods that make up a plant-based diet, they're always struck by how little there is to learn. However, this is most likely due to the removal of many of the meat options. It seems as if a significant portion of the diet has been eliminated as a result of it. How will life be enjoyable without a delicious steak? What are we going to do if we don't have chicken wings? Is there anything that can be achieved in the absence of a tasty fish?

In fact, there are a variety of ingredients with which you can experiment. Furthermore, the fun is not only in the ingredients, but also in the way we prepare them. As a result of the increased demand, more people are trying out new recipes and combining ingredients in novel ways. Have you ever heard of cayenne pepper smoothies? Doesn't it sound like a lot of fun? We'll look at a variety of wonderful and delectable recipes, as well as a variety of other dishes made with wholesome and natural ingredients.

Some people are following it; others are learning about it, but there is still a lot of misunderstanding about what a complete plant-based diet means. Most of us are unsure about nutrition because we divide food into its macronutrients: sugars, proteins, and fats. What if we could reassemble these macronutrients to clear the mind of confusion and stress? The key is to keep things simple. We compile a four-week schedule for you to use over the course of weeks or months.

BREAKFAST RECIPES

1. Banana Waffles

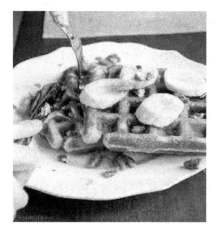

Preparation Time: 5 minutes

Cooking time: 5 minutes

Servings: 6

Ingredients:

- 1/4 teaspoon ground nutmeg

- 1 cup cashew milk, unsweetened

- 1 teaspoon ground cinnamon

- 2 1/2 tablespoon cashew butter

- 1/4 teaspoon baking soda

- 1 peeled medium banana

- 1 tablespoon baking powder

- 7 oz all-purpose flour
- 2 tablespoon sugar

Directions:

1. In a blender, add all the Ingredients: on the list, cashew milk, and baking soda first. Blend for a minute until smooth.

2. In a waffle maker, use a spoon to transfer the mixture and cook the batter over medium-high heat. Your machine might not tell you when they are ready. Take them off when you can no longer see steam.

Nutrition: Calories: 200 Carbs: 35g Protein: 4g Fat: 5g

2. Ginger Chocolate Oats

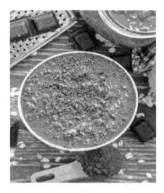

Preparation Time: 3 minutes

Cooking time: 0 minutes

Servings: 1

Ingredients:

- 2 tablespoon chocolate chips
- 1 ¾ oz rolled oats
- 1 cup almond milk
- 1 tablespoon cocoa
- 1/2 teaspoon ground ginger
- 1 tablespoon chia seeds
- 1 tablespoon maple syrup

Directions:

1. In a sealable jar or container, place all fixings; put the milk last. Stir the mixture properly and cover. With the

jar covered, shake properly to mix the fixings. Keep the jar refrigerated for about 6 hours.

Nutrition: Calories: 347 Carbs: 56g Protein: 17g Fat: 12g

3. Gluten Free Pancakes

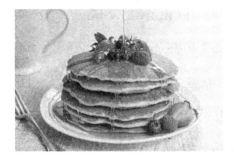

Preparation Time: 10 minutes

Cooking time: 5 minutes

Servings: 6

Ingredients:

- 1 cup almond milk, unsweetened
- 1 filled cup cornflour
- 4 teaspoon vanilla extract
- 1 tablespoon baking powder
- 4 teaspoon sugar
- 1/2 teaspoon salt
- Vegan butter

Directions:

1. In a medium bowl, place baking powder, sugar, cornflour, and salt. Using a whisk, mix these Ingredients: properly.

2. Next, add milk and vanilla to the bowl and continue mixing. Place a skillet over medium-low heat—grease pan with vegan butter. Add the contents of your bowl to the skillet, a third of a cup at a time.

3. Cook each side for about 2 minutes. The sides of the pancakes should be set, and bubbles should be noticeable on top.

4. Use a spatula and be gentle when flipping the pancakes. Take them from the pan, and they're ready to serve.

Nutrition: Calories: 95 Carbs: 19g Protein: 1/2g Fat: 1.3

4. Apple Cinnamon Smoothie

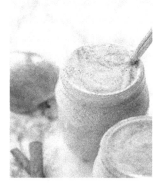

Preparation Time: 5 minutes

Cooking time: 0 minutes

Servings: 1

Ingredients:

- 1 tablespoon flaxseed, ground

- 8 oz coconut water

- 1/2 tablespoon protein powder, unsweetened

- 4 raw almonds

- 1 cup apple, diced

- 1 teaspoon vanilla extract

- 1 teaspoon ground cinnamon

Directions:

1. In your blender, add all fixings. Puree for 15 seconds. Pour into a cup and add 3 cubes of ice.

Nutrition: Calories: 238 Carbs: 37.6g Protein: 15.6g Fat: 5g

5. Pineapple Coconut Mojito Smoothie

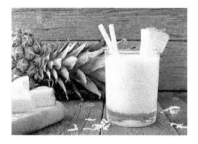

Preparation Time: 5 minutes

Cooking time: 0 minutes

Servings: 1

Ingredients:

- Some ice
- 1 cup coconut milk, unsweetened
- 1 teaspoon chia seeds
- 1/2cup lacinato kale, remove the stems
- 1 tablespoon Sibu Omega-7 Pure
- 1/2 cup spinach leaves, packed
- 1/2 inch piece fresh ginger, peeled
- 1 tablespoon vanilla
- 1/3 cup mint leaves
- 1 cup pineapple chunks, frozen
- 1 lime, peeled, and rind removed

Directions:

1. Put every ingredient except ice in your blender. Puree until a smooth mixture.

2. Add ice cubes and blend once more. Pour into a glass and enjoy.

Nutrition: Calories: 313 Carbs: 30g Protein: 35g Fat: 9g

6. Carrot Cake Quinoa Flake Protein Loaf

Preparation Time: 9 minutes

Cooking time: 6 minutes

Servings: 2

Ingredients:

- 1/2 cup quinoa flakes
- 1/2 cup grated carrots
- 1 1/2 tablespoon protein powder
- 1 teaspoon orange zest
- Pinch salt
- 1/2 cup almond milk, unsweetened
- 4 packets natural sweetener of choice
- 1/3 cup applesauce, unsweetened
- 1 teaspoon ground cinnamon

Directions:

1. In a mini loaf pan, coat with cooking spray. In a medium-sized bowl, add the natural sweeteners, carrots, cinnamon, zest, applesauce, salt, and almond milk. Stir the fixings well.

2. Add protein powder and quinoa flakes. Stir well to incorporate them into the other fixings before putting

the entire batter into the loaf pan. Pat the top to make it even.

3. Cook in the microwave within 6 minutes. Your dessert is ready when the top is firm. Set aside to cool before serving.

Nutrition: Calories: 165 Carbs: 26g Protein: 9.5g Fat: 2.5g

7. Skinny Peanut Butter Protein Smoothie Bowl

Preparation Time: 3 minutes

Cooking time: 0 minutes

Servings: 1

Ingredients:

- Granola of your preference
- 3/4 cup almond milk, unsweetened
- 1 tablespoon protein powder
- 1 tablespoon peanut butter
- 6 ice cubes
- 1/2 cup blueberries, frozen

Directions:

1. Except for the granola, add every ingredient in order into a blender and puree until smooth. Pour the blended mixture into a bowl. Add the granola as a topping.

Nutrition: Calories: 283 Carbs: 21g Protein: 22g Fat: 13g

8. Mocha Smoothie

Preparation Time: 5 minutes

Cooking time: 0 minutes

Servings: 2

Ingredients:

- 2 teaspoon instant espresso powder
- 2 bananas, frozen
- 1 tablespoon cocoa powder
- 1 1/2 cup soy milk

Directions:

1. Add every ingredient on the list into a blender and puree until you get a smooth mixture. Enjoy!

Nutrition: Calories: 114 Carbs: 29g Protein: 2g Fat: 1g

9. Chocolate Peanut Butter Protein Shake

Preparation Time: 5 minutes

Cooking time: 0 minutes

Servings: 1

Ingredients:

- 2 tablespoon hemp hearts
- 1 cup chocolate almond milk
- 1/4 cup peanut butter
- 2 bananas, frozen and finely minced

Directions:

1. Get a blender and throw all the Ingredients: listed above in it. Blend well until smooth.

Nutrition: Calories: 396 Carbs: 68g Protein: 14g Fat: 11g

10. Breakfast Burritos

Preparation Time: 10 minutes

Cooking time: 20 minutes

Servings: 1

Ingredients:

- 4 tortillas, large or burrito size
- 1 cup sliced potatoes
- 1/2 cup salsa of choice
- 1 cup nopales, minced
- Cilantro leaves, roughly diced
- 1 cup black beans, rinse and drain them
- 1 cubed avocado
- 12 oz tofu, extra firm
- Pepper, freshly ground
- Garlic
- Sea salt
- 1 teaspoon ground cumin

Directions:

1. You'll need two saucepans. Set to medium-high heat and add equal amounts of coconut oil to both pans (1 tablespoon) to let them heat.

2. To one pan, add slices of potatoes. Into the other, put the minced nopales. Sauté both.

3. The potatoes should turn a golden color, while the nopales become dry, tender, and turn a brownish color.

4. Shift your nopales to a side of the pan and add tofu. Break the tofu down using a potato masher and keep cooking. You want the tofu to turn brown too.

5. You can add the sautéed potatoes to the pan of nopales now. Also, add black beans, pepper, cumin, salt, and garlic to the pan. Stir and let the mixture cook for 5 minutes.

6. Warm your salsa of choice and tortillas. Cover the mixture in your pan, alongside your salsa and avocado with the tortillas.

Nutrition: Calories: 411 Carbs: 51g Protein: 20g Fat: 14g

LUNCH

11. Asian Flavored Seitan

Preparation Time: 10 Minutes

Cooking Time: 20 Minutes

Servings: 6

Ingredients:

For the seitan:

- 1 ½ tbsp. Vegetable Oil
- 1 lb. Seitan, cubed into 1-inch pieces

For the sauce:

- 2 tsp. Vegetable Oil
- 2 tsp. Cornstarch
- ½ tsp. Garlic, grated
- 2 tbsp. Cold Water
- 1/3 tsp. Red Pepper Flakes
- ½ tsp. Ginger, grated
- ½ cup Coconut Sugar
- ½ cup Vegetable Broth
- ½ cup Soy Sauce

Directions:

1. For making this tasty Asian fare, you need to heat a medium-sized skillet over medium-high heat. To this, spoon in the oil and once it becomes hot, stir in the garlic and ginger while stirring it continuously for half a minute.

2. Then, add red pepper flakes to it and sauté for another one minute or until aromatic. Next, pour the soy sauce and coconut sugar into the mixture. Mix well.

3. Now, lower the heat to medium-low and allow it to simmer for 7 minutes or until the sugar has completely dissolved.

4. Combine the cornstarch and water in another bowl until mixed well, and then pour this into the skillet. Combine.

5. Cook for another 3 minutes and lower the heat to low. Allow the mixture to simmer within 3 minutes or until the sauce is glossy and thickened. Tip: Keep simmering until the seitan gets added.

6. Heat the oil in a medium-sized saucepan over medium-high heat, and to this, add the seitan. Cook them for 5 minutes or until lightly browned.

7. Finally, add the seitan to the sauce and gently toss so that the seitan coats the sauce well. Garnish with sesame seeds and scallions.

Nutrition: Calories: 324 Proteins: 29g Carbohydrates: 33g Fat: 8g

12. Vegan BLT

Preparation Time: 10 Minutes

Cooking Time: 20 Minutes

Servings: 6

Ingredients:

- 3 ½ oz. Tempeh
- ¼ of 1 Avocado, mashed
- 1 ½ tbsp. Tamari
- 1 Tomato, sliced thinly
- 2 tsp. Liquid Smoke
- 1 tsp. Hot Sauce
- 2 slices of Sourdough Bread
- Few Salad leaves
- 2 tsp. Vegan Mayonnaise

Directions:

1. Begin by marinating the tempeh in tamari and liquid smoke. Set it aside for a few minutes. After that, heat the oil in a medium-sized saucepan over medium-high heat.

2. Once the oil becomes hot, stir in the tempeh and fry them for 2 to 3 minutes or golden brown color and slightly crispy.

3. Next, spoon in the marinade over the tempeh and toss well. Then, toast the bread. Now, spread the combo of hot sauce and vegan mayonnaise on one side of the sourdough bread slice.

4. Spread your mashed avocado on the other slice. Finally, layer the bread with the tempeh, salad leaves, and tomato.

Nutrition: Calories: 503 Proteins: 30.9g Carbohydrates: 54g Fat: 21.1g

13. Taco Salad

Preparation Time: 10 Minutes

Cooking Time: 30 Minutes

Servings: 2

Ingredients:

For the taco meat:

- ½ cup Walnuts, soaked for few hours
- ½ tsp. Cumin Powder
- 1 ½ tsp. Chili Powder
- Sea Salt, as needed
- Cayenne Pepper, as needed

For the cashew cream:

- 1 cup Cashews, soaked for few hours
- 3 tbsp. Lemon Juice
- 12 tbsp. Water
- Sea Salt, as needed

For the guacamole:

- 1 Avocado, large & ripe
- ½ tsp. Cumin, grounded
- ¼ cup Red Onion, chopped

- Sea Salt, as needed
- ½ of 1 Tomato, small
- 1 tbsp. + 1 tsp. Lemon Juice

For salad:

- Salad Greens, as needed
- Salsa, as needed

Directions:

1. First, for the taco meat, place all the ingredients in a high-speed blender and pulse them for 20 to 25 seconds or until combined.
2. After that, blend the sauce ingredients in the blender and blend until you get a smooth and creamy sauce.
3. Then, with a fork, mash the avocado in a bowl and, once mashed, stir in the guacamole's remaining ingredients. Mix well.
4. Finally, to serve, place the salad greens on the bottom. On to it top place ¼ of the guacamole in the center.
5. Then, add salsa and half of the taco meat. Pipe the cashew cream over the taco meat. Garnish with green onions if desired.

Nutrition: Calories: 608 Proteins: 11g Carbohydrates: 18g Fat: 59.8g

14. Black Bean Chili

Preparation Time: 10 Minutes

Cooking Time: 30 Minutes

Servings: 6

Ingredients:

- 2 Sweet Potatoes, small & chopped
- 2 Garlic cloves, minced
- 15 oz. Diced Tomatoes
- 1 Onion, small & diced
- 1 tbsp. Chili Powder
- 2 tbsp. Olive Oil
- 15 oz. Black Beans
- 2 Carrots, medium & sliced
- ½ tsp. Garlic Powder
- ½ cup Vegetable Broth
- ¼ tsp. Black Pepper
- 1 tsp. Cumin
- ½ tsp. Salt
- ½ tsp. Cayenne

Directions:

1. First, heat oil in a Dutch oven over medium-high heat. Once the oil becomes hot, stir in the onion and garlic. Mix.

2. Cook them for 3 to 4 minutes or until softened. After that, stir in the sweet potato and carrots to it. Combine.

3. Continue cooking the sweet potato-onion mixture for another 5 minutes or until the veggies soften. Now, lower the heat to low and stir in all the remaining ingredients to the Dutch oven.

4. Give a good stir and cover it partially. Allow it to simmer for 23 to 25 minutes or until everything is cooked. Serve it hot.

Nutrition: Calories: 384 Proteins: 19g Carbohydrates: 67g Fat: 6g

15. Mexican Vegan Casserole

Preparation Time: 10 Minutes

Cooking Time: 30 Minutes

Servings: 8 to 10

Ingredients:

- 3 Tomatoes, chopped
- 1 ½ cups Red Bell Pepper, chopped
- 2 cups Onion, fresh
- ¾ cup of Salsa
- 2 × 15 ¾ oz. Black Beans washed & drained
- Corn Tortillas, needed
- 2 cloves of garlic, minced
- 2 tsp. Cumin, grounded
- 2 cups Vegan Cheese

Directions:

1. For making this tasty casserole fare, preheat the oven to 350 F. After that, heat onion, cumin, pepper, salsa, garlic, and black beans in a large-sized saucepan over medium-high heat.

2. Now, allow the mixture to simmer for 3 to 5 minutes while stirring it frequently. Next, place the corn tortillas on the bottom of a baking casserole.

3. Spoon half the bean mixture over it and then with the vegan cheese. Continue the layering until all are used.

4. Finally, cover the baking dish with a lid and bake for 10 to 15 minutes. Garnish with tomatoes and salsa.

Nutrition: Calories: 595 Proteins: 19g Carbohydrates: 72g Fat: 21g

16. Avocado, Spinach, and Kale Soup

Preparation time: 10 minutes

Cooking time: 0 minutes

Servings: 4

Ingredients:

- 2 avocados, pitted, peeled, and cut in halves
- 4 cups vegetable stock
- 2 tablespoons cilantro, chopped
- Juice of 1 lime
- 1 teaspoon rosemary, dried
- ½ cup spinach leaves
- ½ cup kale, torn
- Salt and black pepper to the taste

Directions:

1. In a blender, combine the avocados with the stock and the other ingredients, pulse well, divide into bowls and serve for lunch.

Nutrition: Calories 300 Fat 23g Carbs 6g Protein 7g

17. Curry Spinach Soup

Preparation time: 10 minutes

Cooking time: 0 minutes

Servings: 4

Ingredients:

- 1 cup almond milk
- 1 tablespoon green curry paste
- 1 pound spinach leaves
- 1 tablespoon cilantro, chopped
- Salt and black pepper to the taste
- 4 cups veggie stock
- 1 tablespoon cilantro, chopped

Directions:

1. In your blender, combine the almond milk with the curry paste and the other ingredients, pulse well, divide into bowls and serve for lunch.

Nutrition: Calories 240 Fat 4g Carbs 6g Protein 2g

18. Arugula and Artichokes Bowls

Preparation time: 5 minutes

Cooking time: 0 minutes

Servings: 4

Ingredients:

- 2 cups baby arugula
- ¼ cup walnuts, chopped
- 1 cup canned artichoke hearts, drained & quartered
- 1 tablespoon balsamic vinegar
- 2 tablespoons cilantro, chopped
- 2 tablespoons olive oil
- Salt and black pepper to the taste
- 1 tablespoon lemon juice

Directions:

1. Combine the artichokes with the arugula, walnuts, and the other ingredients in a bowl, toss, divide into smaller bowls and serve for lunch.

Nutrition: Calories 200 Fat 2g Carbs 5g Protein 7g

19. Minty Arugula Soup

Preparation time: 5 minutes

Cooking time: 10 minutes

Servings: 4

Ingredients:

- 3 scallions, chopped
- 1 tablespoon olive oil
- ½ Cup coconut milk
- 2 cups baby arugula
- 2 tablespoons mint, chopped
- 6 cups vegetable stock
- 2 tablespoons chives, chopped
- Salt and black pepper to the taste

Directions:

1. Heat-up a pot with the oil over medium-high heat, add the scallions, and sauté for 2 minutes. Add the rest of the ingredients, toss, bring to a simmer and cook over medium heat for 8 minutes more. Divide the soup into bowls and serve.

Nutrition: Calories 200 Fat 4g Carbs 6g Protein 10g

20. Spinach and Broccoli Soup

Preparation time: 10 minutes

Cooking time: 20 minutes

Servings: 4

Ingredients:

- 3 shallots, chopped
- 1 tablespoon olive oil
- 2 garlic cloves, minced
- ½ pound broccoli florets
- ½ pound baby spinach
- Salt and black pepper to the taste
- 4 cups veggie stock
- 1 teaspoon turmeric powder
- 1 tablespoon lime juice

Directions:

1. Heat-up a pot with the oil over medium-high heat, add the shallots and the garlic, and sauté for 5 minutes.
2. Add the broccoli, spinach, and the other ingredients, toss, bring to a simmer and cook over medium heat for 15 minutes. Ladle into soup bowls and serve.

Nutrition: Calories 150 Fat 3g Carbs 3g Protein 7g

DINNER

21. The Medi-Wrap

Preparation time: 5 minutes

Cooking time: 0 minutes

Servings: 6

Ingredients:

- ¼ cup crispy chickpeas
- ¼ cup cherry tomatoes halved
- Handful baby spinach
- 2 romaine lettuce leaves, for wrapping
- 2 tablespoons lemon juice, fresh
- ¼ cup hummus
- 2 tablespoons kalamata olives, quartered

Directions:

1. Take a bowl and mix in all ingredients except hummus and lettuce leaves, stir well. Put hummus over lettuce leaves, top with the chickpea mixture. Wrap them up and serve. Enjoy!

Nutrition: Calories: 55 Fat: 0g Carbohydrates: 12g Protein: 3g

22. Nectarine and Quinoa

Preparation time: 15 minutes

Cooking time: 1 hour & 15 minutes

Servings: 6

Ingredients:

- ½ cup kale, chopped
- 1/3 cup pumpkin seeds, roasted
- 3 tablespoons lemon vinaigrette
- 1/3 cup scallions, sliced thin
- 1 cup quinoa, cooked and room temperature
- 2 nectarines, chopped into ½ inch wedges
- ½ cup white cabbage, shredded

Directions:

1. Take a bowl and add all listed ingredients, stir well. Serve and enjoy!

Nutrition: Calories: 400 Fat: 18g Carbohydrates: 52g Protein: 11g

23. Grilled Sprouts and Balsamic Glaze

Preparation time: 15 minutes

Cooking time: 30 minutes

Servings: 2

Ingredients:

- ½ pound Brussels sprouts, trimmed and halved
- Fresh cracked black pepper
- 1 tablespoon olive oil
- Sunflower seeds to taste
- 2 teaspoons balsamic glaze
- 2 wooden skewers

Directions:

1. Take wooden skewers and place them on a large piece of foil. Place sprouts on the skewers and with drizzle oil, sprinkle sunflower seeds and pepper. Cover skewers with foil.

2. Pre-heat your grill to low and place skewers (with foil) in the grill. Grill for 30 minutes, making sure to turn after every 5-6 minutes. Once done, uncover and drizzle balsamic glaze on top.

Nutrition: Calories: 440 Fat: 27g Carbohydrates: 33g Protein: 26g

24. Green Creamy Cabbage

Preparation time: 15 minutes

Cooking time: 10 minutes

Servings: 4

Ingredients:

- 2 ounces almond butter
- 1 and ½ pounds green cabbage, shredded
- 1 and ¼ cups of coconut cream
- Sunflower seeds and pepper to taste
- 8 tablespoons fresh parsley, chopped

Directions:

1. Put almond butter in a skillet over medium heat, and let it melt. Add cabbage and sauté until browns.
2. Stir in cream and turn down the heat to low. Let it simmer. Season with sunflower seeds and pepper. Garnish with parsley and serve. Enjoy!

Nutrition: Calories: 432 Fat: 42g Carbohydrates: 8g Protein: 4g

25. Rice Mushroom Risotto

Preparation time: 15 minutes

Cooking time: 15 minutes

Servings: 4

Ingredients:

- 4 and ½ cups cauliflower, riced
- 3 tablespoons coconut oil
- 1-pound Portobello mushrooms, thinly sliced
- 1-pound white mushrooms, thinly sliced
- 2 shallots, diced
- ¼ cup organic vegetable broth
- Sunflower seeds and pepper to taste
- 3 tablespoons chives, chopped
- 4 tablespoons almond butter
- ½ cup kite ricotta/cashew cheese, grated

Directions:

1. Pulse cauliflower florets using a food processor until rice. Take a large saucepan and heat up 2 tablespoons of oil over a medium-high flame.

2. Put mushrooms and sauté for 3 minutes until mushrooms are tender. Clear saucepan of mushrooms and liquid and keep them to one side.

3. Add the last tablespoon of oil to the skillet. Toss shallots and cook for 60 seconds. Add cauliflower rice, stir for 2 minutes until coated with oil.

4. Add broth to riced cauliflower and stir for 5 minutes. Remove pot from heat and mix in mushrooms and liquid.

5. Add chives, almond butter, and ricotta/cheese. Season with sunflower seeds and pepper. Serve and enjoy!

Nutrition: Calories: 438 Fat: 17g Carbohydrates: 15g Protein: 12g

26. Almond and Blistered Beans

Preparation time: 15 minutes

Cooking time: 20 minutes

Servings: 4

Ingredients:

- 1-pound of fresh green beans ends trimmed
- 1 and ½ tablespoons olive oil
- ¼ teaspoon sunflower seeds
- 1 and ½ tablespoons fresh dill, minced
- Juice of 1 lemon
- ¼ cup crushed almonds
- Extra sunflower seeds as needed

Directions:

1. Preheat your oven to 400degree Fahrenheit. Add in the green beans with your olive oil and also with sunflower seeds.
2. Then spread them in one single layer on a large-sized sheet pan. Roast it up for 10 minutes and stir it nicely, then roast for another 8-10 minutes

3. Remove it from the oven and keep stirring in the lemon juice alongside the dill. Top it with crushed almonds and some sunflower seeds and serve

Nutrition: Calories: 347 Fat: 16g Carbohydrates: 6g Protein: 45g

27. Tomato Platter

Preparation time: 2-3 hours & 15 minutes

Cooking time: 0 minutes

Servings: 8

Ingredients:

- 1/3 cup olive oil
- 1 teaspoon sunflower seeds
- 2 tablespoons onion, chopped
- ¼ teaspoon pepper
- ½ a garlic, minced
- 1 tablespoon fresh parsley, minced
- 3 large fresh tomatoes, sliced
- 1 teaspoon dried basil
- ¼ cup red wine vinegar

Directions:

1. Take a shallow dish and arrange tomatoes in the dish. Add the rest of the ingredients in a mason jar, cover the jar and shake it well. Pour mix over tomato slices. Let it chill for 2-3 hours. Serve!

Nutrition: Calories: 350 Fat: 28g Carbohydrates: 10g Protein: 14g

28. Garbanzo and Spinach Beans

Preparation time: 15 minutes

Cooking time: 0 minutes

Servings: 4

Ingredients:

- 1 tablespoon olive oil
- ½ onion, diced
- 10 ounces spinach, chopped
- 12 ounces garbanzo beans
- ½ teaspoon cumin

Directions:

1. Take a skillet and add olive oil, let it warm over medium-low heat. Add onions, garbanzo and cook for 5 minutes. Stir in spinach, cumin, garbanzo beans and season with sunflower seeds

2. Use a spoon to smash gently. Cook thoroughly until heated, enjoy!

Nutrition: Calories: 90 Fat: 4g Carbohydrates:11g Protein:4g

29. Curried Apple

Preparation time: 15 minutes

Cooking time: 1 hour & 20 minutes

Servings: 4

Ingredients:

- 1 tablespoon fresh lemon juice
- ½ cup of water
- 2 apples, Fuji or Honeycrisp, cored and thinly sliced into rings
- 1 teaspoon curry powder

Directions:

1. Warm your oven to 200 Fahrenheit, take a rimmed baking sheet and line with parchment paper. Take a bowl and mix in lemon juice and water, add apples and soak for 2 minutes.
2. Pat them dry and arrange in a single layer on your baking sheet, dust curry powder on top of apple slices.
3. Bake within 45 minutes, after 45 minutes, turn the apples and bake for 45 minutes more. Let them cool for extra crispiness, serve and enjoy!

Nutrition: Calories: 240 Fat: 13g Carbohydrates: 20g Protein: 6g

30. Cilantro and Avocado Platter

Preparation time: 15 minutes

Cooking time: 0 minutes

Servings: 6

Ingredients:

- 2 avocados, peeled, pitted and diced
- 1 sweet onion, chopped
- 1 green bell pepper, chopped
- 1 large ripe tomato, chopped
- ¼ cup of fresh cilantro, chopped
- ½ a lime, juiced
- Salt and pepper as needed

Directions:

1. Take a medium-sized bowl and add onion, bell pepper, tomato, avocados, lime and cilantro. Mix well and give it a toss. Season with salt and pepper according to your taste. Serve and enjoy!

Nutrition: Calories: 126 Fat: 10g Carbohydrates: 10g Protein: 2g

SNACKS

31. Vegan Fudgy Granola Bar

Preparation time: 15 minutes

Cooking time: 25 minutes

Servings: 16

Ingredients:

- 1 pinch salt
- 1 1/2 cups sliced almonds
- 1/2 cup flaked coconut (unsweetened)
- 1/2 cup pecans
- 1/2 cup sunflower seeds
- 1/2 cup dried, unsweetened cranberries (chopped)
- 1/2 cup butter
- 1/2 cup powdered erythritol
- 1/2 tsp vanilla extract

Directions:

1. With parchment paper line a square baking dish and preheat oven to 300F. In food processor, pulse

sunflower seeds, pecans, coconut, and almonds until crumb like.

2. In a bowl, add pinch of salt and cranberries. Stir in crumb mixture and mix well. In microwave safe mug, melt butter in 20-second interval. Whisk in vanilla extract and erythritol. Pour over granola crumbs and mix well.

3. Press mixture as compact as you can on prepared dish. Pop in the oven and bake for 25 minutes. Let it cool and cut into 16 equal squares.

Nutrition: Calories: 180 Protein: 4.0g Carbs: 5.0gFat: 17.0g

32. Scrumptious Ginger Cookies

Preparation time: 15 minutes

Cooking time: 10 minutes

Servings: 12

Ingredients:

- 1 tsp ground cinnamon
- 1 large organic egg
- 1/2 tbsp ground ginger
- 1/4 tsp sea salt
- 3/4 cup coconut flour
- 3/4 cup unsalted butter (softened)
- 3/4 cup powdered brown sugar erythritol
- 1 1/2 cups almond flour

Directions:

1. Prepare two baking sheets lined using parchment paper and preheat oven to 350oF. In a bowl, whisk well salt, cinnamon, ginger, coconut flour, and almond flour.

2. Add egg and beat well to mix. Knead until you form a dough. Scoop into balls. Roll in powdered erythritol.

3. Place in prepared baking sheet two inches apart. Flatten each cookie and bake until golden brown, around 9 minutes.

Nutrition: Calories: 190 Protein: 3.5g Carbs: 5.5g Fat: 16.0g

33. Cinnamon Muffins

Preparation time: 15 minutes

Cooking time: 15 minutes

Servings: 12

Ingredients:

- 1 tbsp cinnamon
- 1 tsp baking powder
- 1/2 cup almond flour
- 1/2 cup coconut oil
- 1/2 cup almond butter
- 1/2 cup pumpkin puree
- 2 scoops vanilla protein powder

Glaze Ingredients:

- 1 tbsp granulated sweetener of choice
- 2 tsp lemon juice
- 1/4 cup coconut butter
- 1/4 cup milk of choice

Directions:

1. Line 12 muffin tins with muffin liners and preheat oven to 350oF. Whisk well cinnamon, baking powder, and protein powder in a medium bowl.

2. Whisk in coconut oil, almond butter, and pumpkin puree. Mix well. Evenly divide into prepared muffin tins.

3. Bake in the oven for 13 minutes or until cooked through. Move it to a wire rack and let it cool. Meanwhile, mix all glaze ingredients in a small bowl and drizzle over cooled muffin.

Nutrition: Calories: 112 Protein: 5.0g Carbs: 3.0g Fat: 9.0g

34. Vegan Avocado & Spinach Dip

Preparation time: 15 minutes

Cooking time: 0 minutes

Servings: 12

Ingredients:

- 1 garlic clove crushed
- 1 tbsp Extra virgin avocado oil
- 1 tablespoon lime juice
- 1/2 cup fresh spinach leaves in boiling water within 2 minutes, squeezed, drained
- 1/2 teaspoon sea salt
- 1/4 cup fresh coriander chopped
- 2 large ripe avocados about 2 cups of mashed avocado
- 3 tablespoon Extra Virgin Avocado Oil
- 3/4 cup dairy free coconut yogurt

Directions:

1. With paper towel, pat dry blanched spinach leaves. In a blender or food processor, puree pepper, salt, avocado oil, lime juice, coconut yogurt, coriander, crushed garlic, and ripe avocado.

2. Transfer to a bowl and whisk in spinach leaves. Serve and enjoy.

Nutrition: Calories: 91 Protein: 1.1g Carbs: 3.1g Fat: 8.8g

35. Carrot Cake Balls

Preparation time: 15 minutes

Cooking time: 0 minutes

Servings: 15

Ingredients:

- 1/2 cup coconut flour
- 1/2 cup + 1 tbsp water
- 2 tbsp unsweetened applesauce
- 1/2 tsp vanilla extract
- 1 tsp cinnamon
- 4 tbsp Lakanto Classic Monk Fruit Sweetener
- 1 medium carrot, finely chopped or shredded
- 4 tbsp reduced fat shredded coconut

Directions:

1. In a mixing bowl, whisk well vanilla extract, applesauce, water, and coconut flour. Stir in shredded carrots, Lakanto, and cinnamon. Mix well.

2. Place dough in fridge for 15 minutes. Place shredded coconut in a bowl. Evenly divide dough into 15 equal parts and roll into balls.

3. Roll balls in bowl of shredded coconut. Store in lidded containers and enjoy as a snack.

Nutrition: Calories: 24 Protein: 1.0g Carbs: 3.0g Fat: 1.0g

36. Hearts of Palm & Cheese Dip

Preparation time: 15 minutes

Cooking time: 25 minutes

Servings: 9

Ingredients:

- ¼ cup mayonnaise
- ¼ cup Parmesan cheese, for topping
- ½ cup Parmesan cheese, shredded
- 1 (14-ounce) can hearts of palm, drained
- 2 large organic eggs, separate 1 of the eggs
- 2 tablespoons Italian seasoning
- 3 stalks green onions, chopped

Directions:

1. Oiled a small baking dish with cooking spray and preheat oven to 350F. In food processor, add hearts of palm, mayo, Parmesan cheese, seasoning, and green onions. Process until chopped thoroughly.

2. Add 1 egg yolk and one whole egg. Pulse four times. Pour mixture into prepared dish. Pop in the oven and bake within 20 minutes.

3. Remove from oven and mix. Top with cheese. Return to oven and broil until tops are golden brown, around 2 to 3 minutes.

Nutrition: Calories: 74 Protein: 4.9g Carbs: 4.2g Fat: 9.2g

37. Roasted Almonds

Preparation Time: 5 minutes

Cooking Time: 10 minutes

Servings: 16

Ingredients:

- 2 cups whole almonds
- 1 tablespoon chili powder
- ½ teaspoon ground cinnamon
- ½ teaspoon ground cumin
- ½ teaspoon ground coriander
- Salt
- ground black pepper, to taste
- 1 tablespoon olive oil

Directions:

1. Warm oven to 350 degrees F. Line a baking dish with a parchment paper. In a bowl, add all ingredients and toss to coat well.

2. Transfer the almond mixture into the prepared baking dish in a single layer. Roast for about 10 minutes, flipping twice in a middle way.

3. Remove then keep aside to cool completely before serving. You can preserve these roasted almonds in an airtight jar.

Nutrition: Calories: 78 Fat: 6.9g Carbohydrates: 2.9g Protein: 2.6g

38. Cheese Biscuits

Preparation Time: 15 minutes

Cooking Time: 15 minutes

Servings: 8

Ingredients:

- 1/3 cup coconut flour, sifted
- ¼ teaspoon baking powder
- Salt, to taste
- 4 organic eggs
- ¼ cup butter, melted and cooled
- 1 cup cheddar cheese, shredded

Directions:

1. Warm oven to 400 degrees F. Line a large cookie sheet with a greased piece of foil. In a large bowl, mix together flour, baking powder, garlic powder, and salt.

2. In another bowl, add eggs and butter and beat well. Add egg mixture into flour mixture and beat until well combined. Fold in cheese.

3. With a tablespoon, place the mixture onto prepared cookie sheets in a single layer. Bake within 15 minutes or until top becomes golden brown.

Nutrition: Calories: 142 Fat: 12.7g Carbohydrates: 0.8g

Protein: 8g

39. Baked Veggie Balls

Preparation Time: 15 minutes

Cooking Time: 25 minutes

Servings: 8

Ingredients:

- 2 medium sweet potatoes, peeled and cubed into ½-inch size
- 2 tablespoons unsweetened coconut milk
- 1 cup fresh kale leaves, trimmed and chopped
- ½ small yellow onion, chopped finely
- 1 teaspoon ground cumin
- ½ teaspoon granulated garlic
- ¼ teaspoon ground turmeric
- Salt
- ground black pepper, to taste
- ¼ cup ground flax seeds

Directions:

1. Warm oven to 400 degrees F. Prepare a baking sheet using parchment paper. In a pan of water, arrange a steamer basket.

2. Put the sweet potato in your steamer basket and steam for about 10-15 minutes. In a large bowl, place the sweet potato and coconut milk and mash well.

3. Add remaining ingredients except for flax seeds and mix until well combined. Make about 1½-2-inch balls from the mixture.

4. Arrange the balls onto the prepared baking sheet in a single layer and sprinkle with flax seeds. Bake for about 20-25 minutes.

Nutrition: Calories: 61 Fat: 2.1g Carbohydrates: 9g Protein: 1.5g

40. Celery Crackers

Preparation Time: 15 minutes

Cooking Time: 2 hours

Servings: 15

Ingredients:

- 10 celery stalks
- 1 teaspoon fresh rosemary leaves
- 1 teaspoon fresh thyme leaves
- 2 tablespoons raw apple cider vinegar
- ¼ cup avocado oil
- Salt, to taste
- 3 cups flax seeds, grounded roughly

Directions:

1. Warm oven to 225 degrees F. Line 2 large baking sheets with parchment paper. In a food processor, add all ingredients except flax seeds and pulse until a puree form.

2. Add flax seeds and pulse until well combined. Transfer the dough into a bowl and keep aside for about 2-3 minutes. Divide the dough into 2 portions.

3. Place 1 portion in each prepared baking sheets evenly. With the back of a spatula, smooth and press the dough to ¼-inch thickness. With a knife, score the squares in the dough.

4. Bake for about 2 hours, flipping once halfway through. Remove from the oven and keep aside to cool on the baking sheet for about 15 minutes.

Nutrition: Calories: 126 Fat: 7.6g Carbohydrates: 7.1g Protein: 4.3g

DESSERT RECIPES

41. Avocado Pudding

Preparation Time: 3 hours

Cooking Time: 0 minute

Servings: 4

Ingredients:

- 1 cup almond milk
- 2 avocados, peeled and pitted
- ¾ cup cocoa powder
- 1 teaspoon vanilla extract
- 2 tablespoons Stevia
- ¼ teaspoon cinnamon
- Walnuts, chopped for serving

Directions:

1. Add avocados to a blender and pulse well. Add cocoa powder, almond milk, Stevia, vanilla bean extract and pulse the mixture well.

2. Pour into serving bowls and top with walnuts. Chill for 2-3 hours and serve!

Nutrition: Calories: 288 Carbs: 34g Fat: 20g Protein: 4g

42. Crispy Almond Biscotti

Preparation time: 20 minutes

Cooking time: 40 minutes

Servings: 18 slices

Ingredients:

- 2 tablespoons ground flaxseeds
- 1/3 cup unsweetened soy milk
- ¼ cup unsweetened applesauce
- ½ teaspoon vanilla extract
- ½ teaspoon almond extract
- ¼ cup almond butter
- ¾ cup maple sugar
- 1 2/3 cups whole-wheat pastry flour
- 2 teaspoons baking powder
- 1 cup slivered almonds
- 2 tablespoons cornstarch
- 2 teaspoons anise seeds
- ½ teaspoon salt, optional

Directions:

1. Warm your oven to 350ºF. Line a baking sheet with parchment paper.

2. Combine the flaxseeds, soy milk, applesauce, vanilla, almond extract, almond butter, and maple sugar in a large bowl. Stir to mix well.

3. Mix in the remaining ingredients and knead the mixture until a stiff dough form.

4. Shape the dough into a 9-inch-long rectangle in the baking sheet. Bake in the preheated oven for 27 minutes or until golden brown.

5. Remove the baking sheet from the oven. Allow to cool within 20 minutes, then slice the loaf into ½-inch-thick slices.

6. Put the biscotti back to the baking sheet and increase the temperature of the oven to 375ºF (190ºC).

7. Bake in the oven within 11 minutes or until crispy. Flip the biscotti halfway through the cooking time. Transfer the biscotti onto a plate and serve.

Nutrition: Calories: 120 Carbs: 16g Fat: 5g Protein: 3g

43. Raisin Oat Cookies

Preparation time: 15 minutes

Cooking time: 8-10 minutes

Servings: 24 cookies

Ingredients:

- 1/3 cup almond butter
- ½ cup maple sugar
- ¼ cup unsweetened applesauce
- 1 teaspoon vanilla extract
- 1/3 cup sorghum flour
- 2/3 cups oat flour
- ½ teaspoon baking soda
- ½ cup raisins
- 1 cup rolled oats
- ½ teaspoon ground cinnamon
- ¼ teaspoon salt, optional

Directions:

1. Warm your oven to 350ºF. Line two baking sheets with parchment paper. Whisk together the almond butter, maple sugar, and applesauce in a large bowl until smooth.

2. Mix in the remaining ingredients and keep whisking until a stiff dough form.

3. Divide and roll the dough into 24 small balls, then arrange the balls in the baking sheets. Keep a little space between each two balls. Bash them with your hands to make them form like cookies.

4. Bake in the preheated oven for 9 minutes or until crispy. Flip the cookies halfway through the cooking time. Remove them from the oven and allow to cool for 10 minutes before serving.

Nutrition: Calories: 115 Carbs: 14g Fat: 6g Protein: 2g

44. Oat Scones

Preparation time: 15 minutes

Cooking time: 22 minutes

Servings: 12 scones

Ingredients:

- 1 teaspoon apple cider vinegar
- ½ cup unsweetened soy milk
- 1 teaspoon vanilla extract
- 3 cups oat flour
- 2 tablespoons baking powder
- ½ cup maple sugar
- ½ teaspoon salt, optional
- 1/3 cup almond butter
- ½ cup unsweetened applesauce

Directions:

1. Warm your oven to 350ºF. Line a baking sheet with parchment paper. Combine cider vinegar and soy milk in a bowl. Stir to mix well. Let stand for a few minutes to curdle, then mix in the vanilla.

2. Combine the flour, baking powder, sugar, and salt (if desired) in a second bowl. Stir to mix well. Combine

the almond butter and applesauce in a third bowl. Stir to mix well.

3. Gently fold the applesauce mixture in the flour mixture, then stir in the milk mixture.

4. Scoop the mixture on the baking sheet with an ice-cream scoop to make 12 scones. Drizzle them with a touch of water.

5. Bake in the preheated oven within 22 minutes or until puffed and lightly browned. Flip the scones halfway through the cooking time.

6. Remove them from the oven and allow to cool for 10 minutes before serving.

Nutrition: Calories: 177 Fat: 6.0g Carbs: 26.6g Protein: 5.4g

45. Crispy Graham Crackers

Preparation time: 30 minutes

Cooking time: 11 minutes

Servings: 12

Ingredients:

- 1½ cups spelt flour, plus additional for dusting
- ½ teaspoon baking soda
- ¼ cup date sugar
- 1 teaspoon ground cinnamon
- ½ teaspoon salt, optional
- 2 tablespoons molasses
- 1 teaspoon vanilla extract
- ¼ cup unsweetened applesauce
- 1 tablespoon ground flaxseeds
- ¼ cup unsweetened soy milk
- 1 tablespoon maple sugar

Directions:

1. Warm your oven to 350ºF. Line a baking sheet with parchment paper.

2. Combine the flour, baking soda, date sugar, ½ teaspoon of the cinnamon, and salt (if desired) in a large bowl. Stir to combine well.

3. Create a well in the middle of your flour mixture, then add the molasses, vanilla, and applesauce to the well. Whisk to combine.

4. Mix in the flaxseeds and soy milk, then knead the mixture to form a smooth dough. Add a dash of water if necessary.

5. On a clean work surface, dust with a touch of flour, then flatten the dough into a 1/8-inch-thick rectangle with a rolling pin on this surface.

6. Cut the dough into 8 equal-sized rectangles to make the crackers, then arrange the crackers on the baking sheet.

7. Sprinkle the crackers with maple sugar and remaining cinnamon. Poke holes into each cracker with a fork.

8. Bake in the preheated oven for 11 minutes or until crispy and golden brown. Flip the crackers halfway through your cooking time.

9. Remove them from the oven and allow to cool for 10 minutes before serving.

Nutrition: Calories: 120 Carbs: 20g Fat: 3g Protein: 2g

46. Overnight Oats

Preparation time: 5 minutes

Cooking time: 5 minutes

Servings: 1

Ingredients:

- ½ cup rolled oats
- 1 tablespoon ground flaxseeds
- 1 tablespoon maple syrup
- ¼ teaspoon ground cinnamon
- Topping Options:
- 1 pear, chopped, and 1 tablespoon cashews
- 1 apple, chopped, and 1 tablespoon walnuts
- 1 banana, sliced, and 1 tablespoon peanut butter
- 1 cup sliced grapes and 1 tablespoon sunflower seeds
- 1 cup berries and 1 tablespoon unsweetened coconut flakes
- 2 tablespoons raisins and 1 tablespoon hazelnuts
- 2 tablespoons dried cranberries and 1 tablespoon pumpkin seeds

Directions:

1. Combine the ground flaxseeds, oats, cinnamon, and maple syrup in a bowl, then pour the water into the bowl to submerge. Stir to mix well.
2. Leave them to soak within at least 1 hour, or overnight, then serve with the topping you choose.

Nutrition: Calories: 244 Fat: 16.0g Carbs: 10.0g Protein: 7.0g

47. Golden Muffins

Preparation time: 15 minutes

Cooking time: 30 minutes

Servings: 6

Ingredients:

- 1 orange, peeled
- 2 tablespoons chopped dried apricots
- 1 carrot, coarsely chopped
- 2 tablespoons almond butter
- ¼ cup unsweetened almond milk
- 2 tablespoons ground flaxseeds
- 3 tablespoons molasses
- ½ teaspoon ground cinnamon
- ¼ teaspoon ground nutmeg
- ½ teaspoon ground ginger
- 1 teaspoon apple cider vinegar
- 1 teaspoon vanilla extract
- ¼ teaspoon allspice
- ¾ cup rolled oats
- ½ teaspoon baking soda
- 1 teaspoon baking powder

- 2 tablespoons raisins
- 2 tablespoons sunflower seeds

Directions:

1. Warm your oven to 350ºF. Prepare a 6-cup muffin tin lined using parchment paper.
2. Add the orange, apricots, carrot, almond butter, almond milk, flaxseeds, molasses, cinnamon, nutmeg, ginger, vinegar, vanilla, and allspice to a food processor and process until creamy and smooth.
3. Add the rolled oats to a blender and pulse until well ground. Combine the ground oat with baking soda and baking powder in a bowl. Stir to mix well.
4. Pour the orange mixture in the oat mixture, then mix in the raisins and sunflower seeds. Stir to mix well.
5. Divide the mixture into the muffin cups, then bake in the preheated oven for 30 minutes or until puffed and lightly browned. Remove them from the oven and allow to cool for 10 minutes before serving.

Nutrition: Calories: 287 Fat: 23.0g Carbs: 17.0g Protein: 8.0g

48. Coconut and Pineapple Pudding

Preparation time: 15 minutes

Cooking time: 30 minutes

Servings: 2

Ingredients:

- 2 tablespoons ground flaxseeds
- 2 cups unsweetened almond milk
- 1 tablespoon maple syrup
- ¼ cup chia seeds
- 1 teaspoon vanilla extract
- 2 tablespoons shredded, unsweetened coconut
- 1 Medjool date, pitted and chopped
- 2 cups sliced pineapple

Directions:

1. Put the flaxseeds, almond milk, maple syrup, chia seeds, and vanilla extract in a bowl. Stir to mix well.

2. Put the bowl in the refrigerator within 20 minutes, then remove from the refrigerator and stir again. Place the bowl back to the refrigerator for 30 minutes or overnight to make the pudding.

3. Mix in the coconut, and spread the date and pineapple on top before serving.

Nutrition: Calories: 513 Fat: 22.9g Carbs: 66.4g Protein: 16.2g

49. Sweet Potato Toast with Blueberries

Preparation time: 15 minutes

Cooking time: 30 minutes

Servings: 10 slices

Ingredients:

- 1 large sweet potato, rinsed and cut into 10 slices
- 20 blueberries
- 2 tablespoons almond butter

Directions:

1. Warm your oven to 350ºF. Put a wire rack on your baking sheet. Arrange the sweet potato slices on the wire rack, then cook in the preheated oven for 15 or until soft.

2. Flip the sweet potato slices for every 5 minutes to make sure evenly cooked. Then toast immediately or store in the refrigerator.

3. To make the sweet potato toast, put the cooked sweet potato slices in a toaster in batches and toast over medium for 15 minutes or until crispy and golden brown. Serve the toast with blueberries and almond butter.

Nutrition: Calories: 374 Fat: 18.1g Carbs: 47.2g Protein: 10.5g

50. No-Bake Green Energy Super Bars

Preparation time: 15 minutes

Cooking time: 0 minutes

Servings: 36 bars

Ingredients:

- 1½ cups pitted dates, soaked in hot water for 5 minutes and drained
- ½ cup roasted, unsalted cashews
- ½ cup raw sunflower seeds
- 2 tablespoons spirulina powder
- ¼ cup carob
- 2 tablespoons unsweetened shredded coconut
- Pinch of salt, optional

Directions:

1. Put the dates in your blender then process to make the date paste. Add the cashews, sunflower seeds, spirulina powder, and carob. Pulse until dough-like and thick.
2. Put the batter in a baking dish lined using parchment paper, then sprinkle with coconut and salt (if desired).

3. Let stand for 5 minutes, then pull the parchment paper with the mixture out of the container and cut the mixture into 36 bars. Serve immediately.

Nutrition: Calories: 1729 Fat: 79.0g Carbs: 231.0g Protein: 33.0g

CONCLUSION

One of the main reason to eat a plant based diet is to live longer. In addition to taking advantage of the numerous health benefits of a whole food plant-based diet, including shedding off excess weight and lowering your risk of heart disease, cancer, diabetes, autoimmune diseases, and other chronic illnesses that are associated with eating meat and other animal products, a vegan diet is also so much better for you overall in terms of your overall health as well. For example, research has shown that vegans have lower rates of diabetes compared to non-vegans. Even obesity is much less prone among vegans than it is among meat-eaters.

Healthy eating is not the only reason people go vegan. Some do it for their concerns over cruelty to animals, while others do it for the health benefits, and some do it to live a more environmentally sustainable lifestyle. There are many reasons why people stop eating meat, and there are many reasons why people stop eating meat altogether. The most important thing about all of these reasons is that there is one diet that enables them. This plant-based diet is the solution to all of these different reasonings because it's a diet that contains all the necessary nutrients you need as a living being without including any of the harmful ingredients that come attached to animal products. The fact that it's a vegan diet is the reason why plants are referred to as "vegetables" in most contexts.

The benefits of a plant-based diet go far beyond just being healthy. A plant-based diet has been shown to have many benefits for the environment as well. As mentioned before, there are many reasons why people become vegan, but one of the main reasons for doing so is their concern for animal abuse. Being a vegan allows you to take direct action against animal cruelty by helping to support organizations that promote ethical treatment of animals and serving on an activist committee.